HINTS ON
HEALTH

FROM THE
VICTORIANS

HINTS ON HEALTH FROM THE VICTORIANS

Summersdale Publishers Ltd
46 West Street
Chichester
West Sussex
PO19 1RP
UK

www.summersdale.com

Printed and bound in China

ISBN: 978-1-84953-244-0

Disclaimer: Readers are strongly advised not to act on the advice contained in this book.

Substantial discounts on bulk quantities of Summersdale books are available to corporations, professional associations and other organisations. For details telephone Summersdale Publishers on (+44-1243-771107), fax (+44-1243-786300) or email (nicky@summersdale.com).

HINTS ON HEALTH

FROM THE VICTORIANS

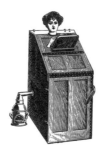

CONSTANCE MOORE

summersdale

Acne, Treatment for

To improve the condition of the blood and general health, take more exercise. To improve a bout of acne, bathe the spots with milk of sulphur. Borax is also good.

Adenoids, Diagnosis of

Children who habitually keep their mouths open to breathe should be examined. If adenoids are found it is best to have them removed while the child is young, as they prevent normal development.

AGUE, CURE FOR

The best way to cure ague
is to hold the feet of a dead
chicken against your body.
[*Ague may refer to fever or malaria.*]

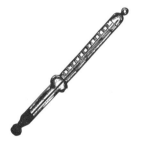

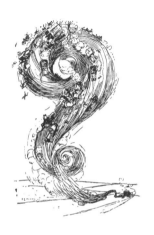

AIR POLLUTION, WAYS TO AVOID

It is well known that infectious
diseases are caused by tainted air.
Everything, therefore, which
tends to pollute the air, or spread
the infection, ought, with the
utmost care, to be avoided.

R. D. Blumenfeld's account of his journey on the Metropolitan underground railway line is testament to this:

'The compartment in which I sat was filled with passengers who were smoking pipes, as is the British habit, and as the smoke and sulphur filled the tunnel, all the windows have to be closed. The atmosphere was a mixture of sulphur, coal dust and foul fumes from the oil lamp above; so that by the time we reached Moorgate Street I was nearly dead of asphyxiation and heat. I should think these Underground railways must soon be discontinued, for they are a menace to health.' (1887)

BALDING, CURE FOR

Rubbing an onion on your head is a very effective cure for baldness.

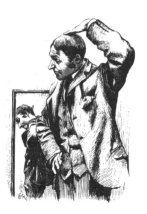

BEE-STINGS AND WASP-STINGS, TREATMENTS FOR

To treat a bee-sting, extract the sting and apply one of the following: moist clay, a blue-bag, bruised rhubarb, ammonia, or moistened baking soda.

To cure a wasp-sting, take the remaining substance from one's smoking pipe and liberally rub it into the aggrieved area.

BLISTERED FEET, CURES FOR

A remedy for blistered feet from long walking is to rub the affected area, on going to bed, with spirits mixed with tallow dropped from a lighted candle into the palm of the hand.

Alternatively, soak your socks in soapy water and leave to dry. Before setting off for the day, add extra protection by cracking a raw egg into the necessary shoes.

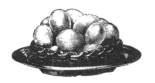

BLUSHING, CURE FOR

To overcome sporadic cases of blushing, take healthy outdoor exercise. Play golf, hockey and tennis, and avoid stuffy or overcrowded places. Sponge the face with oatmeal water, then rinse in cold water to which a little eau-de-Cologne can be added, especially before going in for any excitement. The remedy rests entirely with the patient, who should strive to overcome self-consciousness.

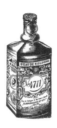

'Oh, yes, yes!' cried Camilla, whose fermenting feelings appeared to rise from her legs to her bosom. 'It's all very true! It's a weakness to be so affectionate, but I can't help it. No doubt my health would be much better if it was otherwise, still I wouldn't change my disposition if I could. It's the cause of much suffering, but it's a consolation to know I possess it, when I wake up in the night.'

Charles Dickens, *Great Expectations*

BODILY POISONS, TO EXTRICATE

Use leeches to withdraw
the 'bad blood' in one's
body. But do avoid overuse
as it could worsen the
initial affliction.

Similarly, take a large quantity of
laxatives to get rid of any bodily
'poisons' through the actions of
both vomiting and diarrhoea.

Bruises, Treatments for

If one is unfortunate enough
to have a nasty fall, rub the
part affected with a piece of
fresh butter, and it will prevent
a bruise from forming, or
any discolouring of skin.

Alternatively, mix two drachms
of bruised opium with half a
pint of boiling water, allow
it to grow cold, and use for
painful ulcers and bruises.

BURNS AND SCALDS, TREATMENTS FOR

Mix as much prepared chalk as you can into some lard, so as to form a thick ointment. Use as an application for burns and scalds.

If the skin is much injured, spread some linen pretty thickly with chalk ointment, and lay over the part. Give the patient some brandy and water if much exhausted; then send for a medical man.

To treat scalds, cover with
scraped raw potato or cover
the parts with treacle, and
dust on plenty of flour.

———•———

A most effective remedy for
burns is to liberally apply cow
dung to the affected area.

Chilblains, Treatments for

Rub every night with oil or cold cream, and sleep in warm socks or stockings.

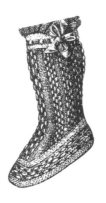

Alternatively, wrap warm, dry, woollen clothing to exposed parts in cold weather, as a preventive. When ulcers form they should be poulticed with bread and water for a day or two, and then dressed with calamine cerate.

CHILDBIRTH, SURVIVING

Ensure that the doctor assisting your birth has clean hands and instruments. This will decrease the risk of fever or death afterwards.

Cholera, Prevention of

The fear of cholera could increase your chances of getting it. Stay calm in its presence.

'Sir,

We live in muck and filth. We ain't got no privez, no dust bins, no water splies and no drain or suer in the whole place. If the Colera comes Lord help us.'

A note to *The Times* newspaper from the poor, 1849

To prevent getting cholera, it is advised to always boil water before using it. The rivers that the water is sourced from are highly polluted and many suppliers take no liability to ensure its cleanliness.

Cholera is also believed to germinate in fruit, vegetables, the sun and a surplus of oxygen. For someone of a superstitious nature, please be aware of your limitations.

COLDS, REMEDIES FOR

I know of no better prophylactic
against colds than the matutinal
tub, cold or tepid, just as a
girl can stand it, only taken
three hundred and sixty-
five times every year, and in
a leap year once oftener.

When benumbed with cold
beware of sleeping out of doors;
rub yourself, if you have it in
your power, with snow, and do
not hastily approach the fire.

COLDS, PREVENTION OF

Those that suffer much from winter's cold should fortify themselves in autumn by taking a two-month course of light brown cod liver oil, and some of the milder preparations of iron.

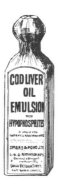

CORNS AND BUNIONS, RELIEF FROM

Bunions may be checked in their early development by binding the joint with adhesive plaster, and keeping it on as long as any uneasiness is felt.

The cause of corns is simply friction, and to lessen the friction you have only to use your toe as you do a coach-wheel – lubricate it with some oily substance.

Cough, Remedies for

To treat a cough, dissolve
three grains of tartar emetic
and fifteen grains of opium in
one pint of boiling water, then
add four ounces of treacle,
two ounces of vinegar and one
pint more of boiling water.

———————

For strengthened effect, mix
alcohol with opium to ease
one's coughing fits. This
remedy also works for those
who are light-sleepers, or are
suffering from loose bowels.

Coughs and Colds,
Treatment for

To make a medicine that will cure both a cough and cold, mix two ounces of solution of acetate of ammonia, two drachms of ipecacuanha wine, two drachms of antimony wine, half a drachm of solution of muriate of morphine, four drachms of treacle; then add eight ounces of water. Two table-spoons must be taken three times a day.

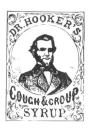

CRAMP, TREATMENT FOR

Stretch out the heel of the leg as far as possible, at the same time drawing up the toes as far as possible. This will often stop a fit of the cramp after it has commenced.

DEPRESSION, HOW TO ALLAY

If one is suffering from depression it is advised to take a sufficient dose of laudanum. Queen Victoria has confirmed the success of this method when she frequently used it to numb the pain of her husband's death.

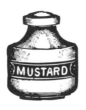

Drunken unconsciousness, Ways to revive from

In the case of unconsciousness from heavy alcohol consumption, raise the head, unloose the clothes; maintain warmth of surface, and give a mustard emetic as soon as the person can swallow.

EARACHE, TREATMENTS FOR

A good sized linseed-meal poultice hot, with eight or ten drops of laudanum in the middle, will cure the most severe earache.

Alternatively, place a ready-cooked baked potato on the painful area and secure tightly. If there isn't one available then a baked onion works just as effectively.

FAINTNESS, TREATMENTS FOR

To treat an instance of faintness, splash one's face in cold water, ensure pure air can travel through the nasal passage and sit the sufferer in the recumbent position. Afterwards, the avoidance of excitement is essential.

To make a 'smelling salt' solution, mix together ammonia and essential oils and pour into a practical bottle to carry around. 'Smelling salts' are most useful to women in the case of short breath from tight corsets. In a situation where one has forgotten their 'smelling salts', try to find the nearest constable as they will specifically carry them around for this purpose.

FISH HOOK OR CROCHET HOOK
IN THE FLESH, TO REMOVE

In the instance of a fish hook or
crochet hook yielding into one's
skin do not attempt to draw it
out. If the accident involves a
child, prevent them doing further
injury by tying their hands,
and seek medical aid at once.

GENERAL ILLNESS, FIGHTING OFF

According to doctors, a good
way to fight off a general illness
is to take a 'healthy' dose of
either mercury, arsenic, iron
or phosphorous. If one has a
strong heart, mix all together.

Persons whose general health is
good bear stronger doses than
the debilitated and those who
have suffered for a long time.

If all medicinal concoctions fail, the next best thing is to pray.

If praying also fails, have the offending limb amputated and hope that the instrument in use has been sterilised well.

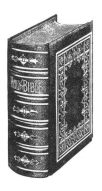

According to the Austrian
doctor, Franz Anton Mesmer,
there are some people who can
heal through look or touch. If
in doubt about your health, find
the nearest healer and endeavour
them to look upon you.

Hay fever, Examination for

Sufferers should be examined by
a surgeon for any defect within
the nose; such is often the cause
of the occurrence of hay fever.

Headaches, Cure for

To cure a headache, sponge
the head all over night and
morning with water as hot
as you can bear it, and rub
dry with a coarse towel.

Place a piece of rock camphor
in a jug of hot water and
inhale the fumes for a
severe cold in the head.

In the fear of one's head
overheating, a well-ventilated
hat will increase the air flow.

Healthy weight, Ways to maintain

Appetite is frequently lost through excessive use of stimulants, food taken too hot, sedentary occupation, costiveness, liver disorder, and want of change of air. The first endeavour should be to ascertain and remove the cause. Change of diet, and change of air, will frequently be found more beneficial than medicines.

The solid part of our bodies is continually wasting, and requires to be repaired by fresh substances. Therefore, food, which is to repair the loss, should be taken with due regard to the exercise and waste of the body.

———•———

Green vegetables contain such valuable medicinal properties that, according to eminent authorities, many of the diseases from which we suffer would be unknown were greens eaten in salad form all the year, instead of being robbed of their precious salts through being boiled in the orthodox wasteful way.

Heart-burn, Treatment for

An agreeable effervescent drink for heart-burn is orange juice. To create the perfect mixture, use one orange, water and a lump of sugar to flavour. To neutralise the acidity of the orange mix in about half a tea-spoon of bicarbonate of soda. Having mixed together the effervescence will ensue.

Home, Ways to improve
the health of

If one lives by a river, it is advised to soak your blinds, or curtains, in chloride of lime to avoid choking on sewage fumes.

We know not of anything
attended with more serious
consequences than that of
sleeping in damp linen.

— ∙ —

Decomposing animal and
vegetable substances yield
various noxious gases, which
enter the lungs and corrupt
the blood. Store away from
rooms that are occupied.

Hysterical fits, Remedy for

Occasional hysterical attacks
need not alarm; the patient
will recover gradually by
herself. Unnecessary fussing
and sympathy often result in
the renewal of an attack.

Irritable bowels, To avoid

To avoid constipation
observe a regular period of
evacuating the bowels, which
is most proper in the morning
after breakfast. Avoid too
much dry and stimulating
food, wine and opium.

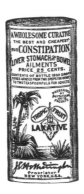

If one suffers from frequent
irritable bowels it is advised
to flush the body by taking
one antimony pellet every
week. Once used and passed
through the body, the pellet
can then be stored away until
necessary to take again.

JAUNDICE, REMEDIES FOR

To cure a case of jaundice mix together one penny-worth of allspice, ditto of flowers of brimstone, ditto of turmeric; these to be well-pounded together, and afterwards to be blended with half a pound of treacle. Two table-spoonfuls to be taken every day.

Lung infections, Relief from

To relieve asthma the following
is recommended: Two ounces
of the best honey, and one
ounce of castor oil mixed.
One tea-spoon must be
taken night and morning.

To prevent consumption
(tuberculosis) one should try to
avoid cold, damp conditions and
excitement, or overexertion.

MALPRACTICES, WARNINGS AGAINST

Lying late is not only hurtful, by the relaxation it occasions, but also by occupying that part of the day at which exercise is most beneficial.

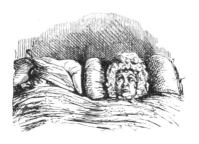

Late hours, irregular habits, and want of attention to diet, are common errors with most young men, and these gradually, but at first imperceptibly, undermine the health, and lay the foundation for various forms of disease in later life.

MASSAGE, AVOIDING

MALPRACTICE OF

Although beneficial in many instances, it is not advisable for any unskilled person to practise massage, though gentle rubbing for pains in the limbs can be applied without much harm being done.

NERVES, TO CALM

To calm the nerves eat a
sandwich twice daily of
caraway seeds, ginger and salt,
spread over buttered bread.

NOSEBLEEDS, REMEDIES FOR

The perfect cure for a
nosebleed is to place a nettle
leaf on your tongue and press
it hard against the roof of your
mouth. If a nettle leaf is not
forthcoming then you should
place a large key against the
skin of the back.

Rheumatism, Cure for

To cure rheumatism, liberally
apply the following concoction
to the area of complaint:
goose grease, horseradish juice,
mustard and turpentine.

Runny nose, Remedy for

To stop one's nose from
running, it is advised to either
sniff an old mouldy sock or a
generous handful of wet salt.
Both of these methods should
effectively clear the airways.
Alternatively, drink hot whisky.

Sexual activity, Warnings against

The experience of sex for many women is an unhappy one that usually leads to pregnancy, along with the fear of death during the birth. The best advice would be to discuss with your partner how many children you want to try to avoid unwanted pregnancies.

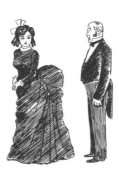

At all costs one must abstain from masturbation. If this rule is violated, women, your hair will fade, your feet will smell and your eyes go dull. If done excessively, this could cause epilepsy, insanity and premature death. Men, you will suffer from blindness and insanity. If done excessively, your genitals will eventually shrink and waste away.

SLEEP DEPRIVATION, PREVENTION OF

The inability to sleep is caused
by blood pressing on the brain.
Insomniacs are overexcited
individuals, often of a nervous
disposition. Brush the body
to promote circulation as this
deliberate chafing will calm
the brain and allow the sufferer
a relaxing night's sleep.

SMOKING, MEDICINAL
ADVANTAGES OF

Tobacco-smoke is a
preventive of malaria.

***

A cigarette, despite it staining
one's teeth, is notably accredited
as a miracle cure for illnesses.

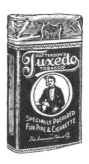

STAYING HEALTHY, HINTS ON

Sir Astley Cooper said, 'The
methods by which I have
preserved my own health
are: temperance, early rising,
sponging the body every
morning with cold water,
immediately after getting out
of bed; a practice which I have
adopted for thirty years without
ever catching cold.'

***

Children should not be forced
to bathe in the sea; the sudden
coldness and action of the salt on
the skin is beneficial to some,
harmful to others.

A sickly person living in London should try to escape to the countryside. With overcrowding, poor sanitation and large poverty-stricken areas, the chances of catching something are elevated.

—◦—

If a person with any ill-related symptoms comes close to you, try not to come into contact with them. A carrier of disease can only be distinguished by their ill, spectral complexion.

STOMACH UPSETS, CURE FOR

To cure an upset tummy
take a pinch of gunpowder,
mix it in a glass of warm
soapy water, and drink.

TEETH, TREATMENTS FOR

To improve stained teeth, a good
scrub with some charcoal is
encouraged to make them whiter.

To allay the pain of a rotten tooth, fill it with a rubber called 'gutta percha' – used mainly to make the core of a golf ball – by boiling until soft and then leaving to set in the desired area.

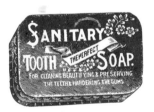

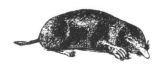

Teething pain, Relief from

To ease the pain of teething,
hang a dead mole around
the neck of your baby.

The sick, Optimum conditions for

The patient's room must be
kept in a perfectly pure state,
and arrangements made for
proper attendance. Keep
the air the patient breathes
as pure as the external air,
without chilling him.

The sick-room should be quiet; no talking, no gossiping, and, above all, no whispering – this is absolute cruelty to the patient; he thinks his complaint the subject, and strains his ear painfully to catch the sound.

It is a good plan to have a card with the word 'Asleep' in large letters written on it, with a ribbon attached to it to hang on the door-handle: it will often prevent the rousing of the patient from a sleep, which is as vexatious to the person who has the misfortune to do so as to the sufferer and the anxious nurse.

VISITORS OF THE SICK,
OPTIMUM CONDITIONS FOR

Do not visit the sick when you
are fatigued, or when in a state of
perspiration, or with the stomach
empty – for in such conditions
you are liable to take the infection.

When the disease is very
contagious, take the side of
the patient which is near to the
window. Do not enter the room
the first thing in the morning
before it has been aired.

WARTS, TO REMOVE

If you are unfortunate enough
to suffer the affliction of warts,
try rubbing half an apple over
the offending protrusion and the
wart should fall off in a few days.

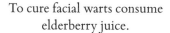

To cure facial warts consume
elderberry juice.

WEATHER, HINTS ON

It is dangerous to stand
about in a cold place with a
light dress. A Shetland shawl
has saved many a life.

———— · ————

There is no better way to protect
freckles from the exposure of
sunlight than to mix together half
a drachm of muriate of ammonia,
two drachms of lavender water
and half a pint of distilled water.
For best effects apply with a
sponge two or three times a day.

If the weather appears doubtful, always take the precaution of having an umbrella when you go out, particularly going to church. The consequence of frequent exposure to unexpected showers, to say nothing of colds taken, is immeasurable.

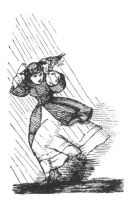

Whooping cough, Remedies for

To cure a bout of whooping cough place a spider in a chunk of butter and swallow in one.

———•———

To rid a child of whooping cough I recommend that the father takes the child to a field at sunset and *gently* holds their head in a hole.

Alternatively, if the child is over ten, the dispensary can offer B. H. Douglass and Sons' Capsicum Cough Drops for all manner of coughs and cold symptoms.

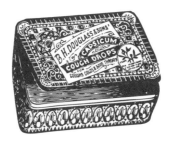

Worms, To remove

The 'Tapeworm Trap', invented by Dr Meyer, has been designed to extricate a tapeworm in the stomach. To do so, take a piece of string and attach to a cylinder filled with food. The patient must then starve themselves and lower the cylinder down into the stomach. Wait until the worm eats from the cylinder, which will automatically trap it, and then the string can be pulled back out.

As an alternative and less painful method, the patient must starve themselves. Then, this must be followed by frying a good batch of bacon. The smell will then diffuse into the pit of the stomach where the worm should immediately jump out of one's mouth from the irresistible temptation to have some.

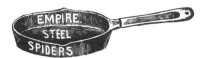

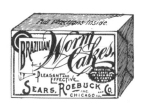

Children suffering from worms may grind their teeth while asleep. Do not give uncooked meat or vegetables, especially watercress, or allow the child to drink unfiltered water. Worm powders or cakes can be procured from any chemist and are quite pleasant to take.

Wrinkles, To remove

Rub cream along the line of the wrinkle – never massage across – after washing the face with warm water, night and morning. Persistent treatment will prove successful, but the cause, such as frowning or twisting the muscles of the face, must be overcome.

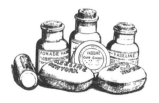

HINTS ON COOKERY

FROM THE VICTORIANS

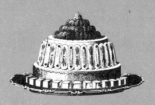

CONSTANCE MOORE

HINTS ON COOKERY FROM THE VICTORIANS

Constance Moore

ISBN: 978 1 84953 246 4   Hardback   £3.99

Cookery is one of the Arts.
Those who would excel in
it must, like other artists,
be educated for it...

For tips on how to be a goddess of domesticity, a modern-day Beeton and a purveyor of familial joy, dive into this miscellany of hints on cookery from the Victorians.

www.summersdale.com